Supercharge Your Health Vibe!

The Supercharge Your Health Vibe Training Course

The inner-world system for your outer-world success.

The scientifically based inner secret of how to feel energized and healthier, even if you have a medical condition or physical limitations!

BY ELIZABETH MENZEL

Book 2 of the Supercharge Your Vibe! series

DISCLAIMER

The material contained in this book was developed from the personal & professional experiences of the author, Elizabeth Menzel. Ms. Menzel is not a mental health professional and makes no claim to be one. She does not make any diagnoses, and she makes no claims to be able to do so.

This book is not intended as a substitute for the advice of and treatment by a qualified physical or mental health professional. The publisher and author are not responsible for any adverse consequences or experiences that may result from the use of the ideas, perspectives, and/or tools discussed in this book.

If you proceed to read and use the material contained in this book, you are accepting responsibility for your actions and the results you create. If you have questions about the efficacy and utility of this material for you, we advise you to consult a health professional or other qualified advisor before implementing the ideas shared here.

DEDICATION

This book is dedicated to you who know what it's like to feel frustrated with your body, drained of energy, and worried that you might not ever feel good again. It's time to align yourself with the vast vitality of the Universe and see what it's like on the other side of an accepting, kind, balanced body and mind. Give this gift to yourself and as you supercharge your health vibe, help others to supercharge theirs.

ALSO BY ELIZABETH MENZEL

Supercharge Your Money Vibe!

WOMEN'S HEALTH BEST-SELLER
Get ready to learn the exact ways I quadrupled my financial income by changing my poverty consciousness to prosperity consciousness as well as how I improved my relationship with money – all while keeping my integrity and working less hours - so that you can do the same for yourself.

Supercharge Your Love Vibe!

WOMEN'S HEALTH BEST-SELLER
Get ready to learn the exact ways I attracted the man of my dreams by changing my broken heart into the well spring of love it's meant to be. As well as how I improved my relationship with my family, my emotions, my body, humanity, and romance, so that you can do the same for yourself.

The 10-Minute Memoir

BEST-SELLER
This book came from a deep heartfelt desire to know the stories of my family. Write Your Memoir In Just 10 Minutes A Day With This Easy Q&A Journal

ABOUT ELIZABETH

Elizabeth Menzel is a certified Brennan Healing Science practitioner and serves as a speaker, best selling author, Happy Woman Mentor, and she's the founder of the award winning Happy Woman Academy. Her books and programs focus on ending the cycle of sacrifice, sabotage, and neglect so that women can enjoy massive success in their career, health, and love life.

She uses proven neuroscience and physics based healing systems and has facilitated thousands of transformations over the last 23 years. Her live events & Happiness Training Programs teach busy women of all ages powerful "on the go" ways to heal their body, invigorate their romance, and boost their career – so they can receive more money while enjoying life more fully! She's on a mission to teach 1,000,000 women "The Happy Woman Formula" by 2020.

The mission of the Happy Woman Academy is to provide women with a safe and sacred space to learn how to easily receive more love, health, and money by using proven science based healing systems and the power of communion and laughter.

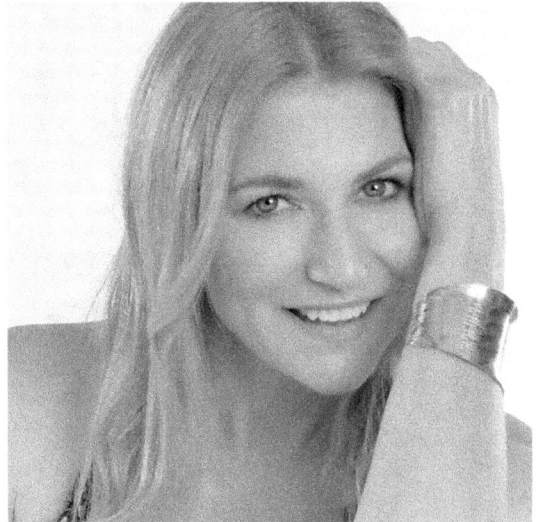

The vision of the Happy Woman Academy is to restore the Feminine to her rightful place of honor & value next to the Masculine in society, thereby restoring harmonic balance to humanity, the earth, & nature. Big vision I know, but it's the one I've got.

CONNECT WITH ME

Visit www.TheHappyWomanAcademy.com/quiz
And take the 30 second quiz to find out the
#1 way you Sabotage Your Success & Happiness

AND

Visit the Happy Woman Academy on Facebook at
https://www.facebook.com/TheHappyWomanAcademy/

AND

I love hearing from my readers, so please feel free to
leave a positive review on my Amazon Author page
at bit.ly/AmazonAuthorElizabethMenzel

CONTENTS

ACKNOWLEDGMENTS

While this book is the culmination of 37 years of personal growth, a decade of dedicated training, and 23 years of professional practice, I didn't do it alone. I'm deeply grateful to my teachers for putting up with my endless questions, to my clients for their dedication to healing and for keeping my skills sharp, and to my dear friends for their care, patience, and riotous laughter. A special thanks to Victor Thompson for cheerfully designing these fabulous book covers and to Stacey & Daniel Canfield at MyImageArtist.com for a magical photo experience.

To Dale Thomas Vaughn, thank you for loving me so completely.

What a special tribe of Vibe Superchargers I have in my life!

Let's all keep Supercharging Our Vibes together!

INTRODUCTION - GET READY

Welcome to Supercharge Your Health Vibe! Get ready to learn my favorite ways I keep my energy strong all day long, feel healthy even when I'm sick or injured, and how I learned to love my body and become the healthiest me I can be, so that you can do the same for yourself.

The training exercises in this book are the missing link for many people who have tried everything, yet have hit a wall they can't move past. If you've spent a lot of time, energy, and money trying to feel better and not feeling as good as you think you could, then these effective inner world solutions could be the key to the outer world success you have been hoping for.

THIS BOOK IS FOR YOU IF:

You are faced with a health challenge.

You have low energy or your energy dips in the day.

You eat right and exercise, but still don't feel great.

You know you should eat right and exercise, but you just can't

seem to do it.

You just don't feel as good as you want to.

You are great at many things, but taking care of your health

isn't one of them.

You get mad at your body.

There is a chance your self esteem could use some boosting.

You feel great, AND YOU WANT TO FEEL EVEN BETTER!

Recently my mother said to me with exasperation, "I'm so tired of taking care of my body all of the time!"

Can you relate? I can! There are so many things you need to do to care for the miraculous body you live in. Cleaning, feeding, hydrating, exercising, moving it from one place to the next, keeping it at a comfortable temperature, resting, playing, sleeping, are the bare minimum things you need to do to maintain good health.

But wait there are more things you need for good health: braces for your teeth, innersoles for your shoes, glasses, medicine, bandages, tissues, a supportive mattress, lotion, vitamins, appliances to cook and store food, ergonomic seating… the list of body care items seems endless. I have 2 bathrooms bursting with products and an impressive herbal apothecary in my kitchen!

Oh my goodness, then there are all of the people that you need to help you maintain good health. I believe a part of staying healthy is relying on a trustworthy "healing team" to support you. I've got an M.D., an acupuncturist, a dentist, a nurse practitioner, an optometrist, several massage therapists, a trainer, a chiropractor, a mentor, 2 support groups, and a fabulous hair stylist on my healing team.

But here is the kicker: all of these great things and people are only half of the solution to great health. True, we all need plenty of outer world help to maintain great health, but you'll never get to the level of health you desire inside of your body without also dealing with your inner world.

I want to change that old saying, "If you don't have your health you don't have anything" to "If you don't have your health you need to supercharge your health vibe."

Would you expect your car to run without gas, water, or oil? No, of course not. Many of you won't go without a haircut, manicure, & new shoes for that special event, but you expect your body to run without enough sleep, exercise, water, and nutrition. Lots of people get stuck in the rut of skimping on the bottom line of good health and even people who don't skimp on the bottom line can get stuck with low energy and health challenges when they don't put the missing piece into place that I'm giving you in this workbook.

I'm not a doctor or nutritionist, so I won't be giving you medical or supplemental advice. I serve as a certified Brennan Healing Science Practitioner and a certified rehabilitative muscle therapist with a 23 year professional practice and have helped thousands of people get well and feel energized. I am a huge advocate of proper nutrition, proper medical care, and medical testing. In fact, I won't even treat my clients for medical issues unless they've had proper medical testing first. Because: 1) I always want you to have the most thorough care possible, 2) holistic medicine includes traditional allopathic medicine, 3) I want you to have quantifiable evidence that the energy healing treatments I give and exercises in this book WORK!   So please, if you are experiencing pain or symptoms that have gone untreated, GO SEE A DOCTOR NOW.

You've got to keep taking all of those great outer world actions you already are doing to improve your health - plus - add in these effective inner world actions and you will start to feel better and supercharge your health vibe! (I mean you've tried everything else you may as well do all of the exercises in this book and see what happens. But watch out, you might have fun doing this!)

A little bit about my health history before we get started on your health transformation. I was raised in a typical working class family in the Lehigh Valley in Pennsylvania. Some early childhood health memories locked in scary beliefs about self-care, physical needs, my looks, my body, and my self worth. As a kid I felt embarrassed and guilty any time I got sick or hurt because I thought that I'd be viewed as weak and I didn't want to be a burden to my mom, so I would often pretend I was fine when I was actually injured or ill. But, I was so stressed out by my parent's divorce and the pressures it put on my mom, that by the 4th grade I missed much of the year of school due to mystery abdominal pain.

Because of stress I had insomnia and stayed up all night, then would be exhausted all day at school, and then sleep all weekend long. I broke so many bones my doctor would just look at me and say, "What did you break this time?" Yikes, it is painful to look back at that scared, nervous little girl that kept getting sick and hurt.

My mom was a big believer in mind over matter, but my young mind converted that concept into, "Ignore it and pretend it's fine and it will go away." And sometimes I actually did think myself well. The mind IS very powerful, but I didn't have a full grasp on my healing capabilities nor was I educated on proper self-care & nutrition.

My mom and I moved to Hollywood, CA when I was 13 years old. I was living on my own by 16 years old and continued ignoring my physical needs, plus I added in ignoring my emotional and mental needs as well. I worked full time but was poor and barely ate. I became a master of denial, highly self sufficient, and utterly clueless of what I needed to do to be truly healthy.

From childhood through young adulthood I felt guilt, fear, undeserving, and embarrassed about my body and I ignored and denied what was going on inside of me. But, I thought I had it all under control.

I liked the idea of taking vitamin supplements and even went vegetarian as a teen and then totally vegan in my 20's. As I became a healer I did a lot of cleanses and fasts, but after years of being vegan I felt totally drained of energy. I was doing so many great things for myself, meditation, massage, chiropractic, exercise, psychotherapy, energy healings, but I just didn't feel good physically and symptoms of depression were getting worse.

Thankfully, through decades of training and receiving therapy and healings, I've found and test driven the most effective self-healing methods. I use them on myself and teach them to thousands of people worldwide. Contained in this workbook are exercises I've used to switch from focusing on what is wrong with me to being able to see my strengths, heal my body, and feel better. I've come a long way: I'm more fit now than 20, even 30 years ago, plus I now have a sense of emotional well being as my baseline, and I have consistent energy all day long.

Over the years I've steadily improved the relationship with my body and I still have room for improvement. I practice supercharging my health vibe regularly and I get extra support from my Happy Woman Academy sisters in our monthly WoManifestation Circles™. I actively use the 5 simple steps in my "Happy Woman Formula" every day and I've compiled 50 of the most effective self-healing exercises that are only available in my "Happy Woman Training Program." I understand that you are busy and might not always have tons of extra time, so most everything I teach helps you to retrain your brain and boost your energy while on the go.

Doing everything on your own is just too hard. It's much more fun to go through life supercharging your health vibe with other fun, supportive, awesome women. That's what the Happy Woman Academy is here for! So, no more going it alone, you are surrounded by allies who want to help you along your healing journey, let us.

No matter what you have been through, you can shed the beliefs that hold you down and move through what holds you back. You can re-wire your brain. You can learn to feel healthier even if you are banged up or have a disease. I've done it, so I know you can do it to.

CHAPTER 1 - DISCOVER YOUR WHY & FIND YOUR MOTIVATION!

Have you ever played with metal tuning forks? If you hold one tuning fork in each hand and hit one of them on something hard the metal vibrates making a sound. Soon the tuning fork that you didn't hit on something hard, that you held perfectly still in your other hand, will start to vibrate and make a sound. This is happening all of the time between you and other people and things, and you are so used to feeling it, that you barely even notice it.

But I bet you have experience it. Have you ever been peacefully sitting there alone reading a book, when suddenly you feel something and can tell someone is standing behind you? Have you ever walked into a room and it just felt good in there? Have you ever been driving the same route home, suddenly decided to make a turn and go a different way, then found out you avoided a huge traffic jam? If you've answered yes to anything even similar to these questions, then you have experienced energetic vibration at work.

And that is because you are made of light, plasma, and sub-atomic particles – in other words, you are made of energy.[1] Energy has a vibration, and that vibration emanates from you - and people and things respond to your vibration, just like the tuning forks. [2][3] So, when you are feeling great, that vibrational wave is sending out a signal from you and you feel in harmony with anything or anyone around you that is also feeling great. When you are feeling happy, it is easier to notice other happy people around you because you are a vibrational match to them. But when you are feeling lousy, you often notice the other people around you that are feeling lousy. If you are complaining in line at the grocery store, there is soon another person complaining right along with you. But often if you are in a good mood at the check out line, people are really nice and helpful. In little and big ways, everything and everyone around you is constantly responding to your vibration and showing you what you are thinking and feeling by how they treat you and what happens to you.

It's time to stop sending out the vibrations that you don't want; that only works to depress your health vibe, hold you back, and keep you from the feeling as good as you could.

In order to maintain good health you have to choose thoughts, words, and actions of healthiness more often than you choose thoughts of unhealthy things. Now you see why it is so important for you to supercharge your health vibe and why you were attracted to getting this book? Yes!

> **Your job is to make yourself the vibrational match to the health that you DO want to have in your life.**

But watch out! Shifting into healthy vibrations can bring up a lot of resistance and fights in your mind, because your mind knows what it is used to feeling as "life" – even if those are feelings you don't like, they are still associated with "Being Alive." So, when you try to change into healthier vibrations, even though they are going to eventually feel better once you get used to them, the mind temporarily registers the new healthy vibration as a threat and equates it to "death." Yes, I'm saying the good health you want can be viewed as so threatening to the old way of life in your mind that you could feel scared enough to give up on trying to feel good.

As you move forward doing the exercises in this workbook that will eventually make you feel healthier, the resisting thoughts could get louder and might sound something like:

"This is dumb. I don't want to do this any more."

"This isn't going to work, I quit."

"I hate this workbook. Forget it."

"I don't believe this stuff. It probably won't work for me anyway."

The act of resisting feeling good zaps your energy and leaves you feeling depleted and exhausted, which makes it difficult for your body to heal. So even if that level of life vs. death resistance comes up while doing this training course, dig deep and gift yourself this full healing experience. These exercises may seem simple on the surface, but take a leap of faith and keep moving forward throughout the whole workbook. These simple actions create change for the better on a deep level within you and on a practical level in your outer world. I've seen this happen for myself and the thousands of people I've helped over the last two decades.

If you need extra motivation and support, you can easily go to TheHappyWomanAcademy.com/quiz and take the quiz to "Find out the #1 way you sabotage your Success & Happiness." This will give you a great jump start plus I'll walk you through a training exercise that you can use to supercharge your health vibe. AND there is an additional bonus at the back of this book waiting to reward you AFTER you complete this workbook. Yes, I really want you to heal so much that I'm willing to give you all of this free help!

Here is a weird question, but it could be holding you back so I have to ask you. Is there a chance that you might feel afraid of feeling happy? It took a lot of conscious awareness before I realized that I was often in a state of "bracing myself" waiting for the other shoe to drop. It used to be more obvious; I spent most of the time feeling a constant un-ease until less than a decade ago. A few years ago I noticed that while the unease had greatly reduced, there was this residual sneaky occasional thought, "If I truly feel happy, something bad will come in to wreck it!" Lately I feel happy and grateful much of the time, yet I notice that I'm still holding myself back from feeling truly fantastic all of the time, so there is still room for improvement. This workbook is going to help you if you suffer from feeling nervous about feeling good.

If you happen to judge feeling happy as "not cool," you're going to have a difficult time manifesting the health you want. You might want to consider letting that limiting belief go and replacing it because it's just blocking the health you want to experience from you, and making you less fun at parties. "Feeling happy is cool." See if you can get behind that belief instead.

Even if you've done this course before, doing it again and again can only help you to supercharge your health vibe. You want this for yourself too much to cheat yourself out of this, so I'm going to trust you to follow the instructions and do each and every training exercise. And if you want extra help beyond this training course, I'm here for you. So go for it, keep building those health muscles! I believe in you, you can do this!

Take a deep breath........... open up your heart and mind & program yourself to get exactly what you need by stating out loud,

> **"I fully engage in this training and get exactly**
> **what I need to supercharge my health vibe."**

Make it official:

Signature_____ Date_____

SETTING YOU UP FOR SUCCESS

It is easy to buy a workbook and then let it sit on a shelf. I want you to have the transformation that you want and that I know you can have. So, you are going to want to make Supercharging Your Health Vibe your priority over the next few weeks.

1.   Success breeds success. Put time to do these training exercises on your calendar.

Only put an amount of time that seems realistic and easy to achieve. Instead of 1 hour a day, how about 10 minutes a day. Or a 1-hour chunk of time twice a week? Then when you do more than that it's a bonus. But if you do less than that you will feel bad and give up. So, put small doable chunks of time on your calendar and give yourself the enormous gifts this book has in store for you.

2.   Stay accountable, get a buddy.

It's way more fun to do a new activity with someone else that you can relate with. You can keep each other motivated and while it can be easier to break a promise to yourself, it's been proven that you keep your word better if you promise someone else you are going to do something. I give you my full permission to share this workbook with a good ally that you can Supercharge Your Health Vibe with, and have fun keeping each other on track and accountable!

3.   Fully Participate.

For you to get the full benefit of this training course you've got to fully participate. You can't just read through it and understand the concepts and think that will do the trick. Just like you have to do weight training to get stronger muscles, you've got to do all of these exercises to train your health vibe to get stronger. But don't worry, it only takes 1 second to start to supercharge your vibration and after just 17 seconds it picks up momentum to become your new normal! So little by little you will keep getting stronger and supercharging your health vibe.

4.   Write it down

Make sure you write your answers to all of the exercises; don't just answer them in your head. Bring thoughts into the material world by writing them down. You can write your answers directly into this book, or if you got it on Kindle you can just write them out in a notebook or a journal.

The main thing is that you DO EVERY EXERCISE COMPLETELY.

We are going to deeply explore then expand your health world. So let's jump right in and get started supercharging your health vibe!

Training Exercise 1-1

I'm sure there are lots of reasons that you want to feel healthier. Go ahead and Write down the TOP 3 things you want good health for:

1. _____

2. _____

3. _____

Training Exercise 1-2

Now get more specific. (If you repeat any of the above reasons, that is ok.) Write down the top reasons why you want to Supercharge Your Health Vibe in each category:

1.   Body: _____

2.   Emotions: _____

3.   Mind: _____

4.   Relationships:_____

5.   Career: _____

6.   Life Vision:_____

7.   Other:_____

Great! Keep referring to this list as you go forward through this training. If you regularly practice what I offer here, you will start to see changes in your health that reflect these lists and that will keep you inspired to continue your training, so that your health vibe grows stronger and stronger.

Training Exercise 1-3

Now, What are the top 3 most valuable things in your life? Write them down quickly without thinking too hard.

1.   _____

2.   _____

3.   _____

Good. Now, look at that list again. Are any of those 3 things money?

Money is a concept that represents value in our society, yet money in and of itself is not A Value. I bring that up right at the beginning because money is so revered in a capitalistic society that people mistakenly replace their personal values with monetary value by judging their worth and importance monetarily. But as you see, the top 3 valuable things in your life aren't all about the Benjamins.

> Your value as a human is not dependent
> on money or achievement.

Are any of these 3 "things" people? Do any of them have to do with Love? I thought so.

Love is the most valuable thing you have to give. Look at how many songs are written about love! Yet, in our society, people mistakenly replace this most precious thing with monetary goals or getting things checked off of their to do list. As if that paperwork, errand, or dirty dishes are more important than kissing your man, hugging your children, or taking care of your health.

> You know love and health are the most valuable things you have,
> so put it in the proper perspective and make
> LOVE & HEALTH FIRST your motto.

To have a healthy relationship with your body, you can't keep feeding it hate with your negative thoughts, words, feelings, and actions. Brain research shows you have to have 5 times more positive thoughts than negative thoughts just to get to neutral.[4] So let's have 10 more positive thoughts about your body, to make sure you supercharge your Health Vibe and starve out all of the negative things you do — probably without even realizing that you are weakening your health.

To gain a new perspective it can help to depersonalize the concept of your health and reframe it simply as an energy. Remember how your top 3 values had something to do with love? What I noticed is that love is an infinite energy. Money, for example, is a finite energy.

Humans are naturally attracted to infinite energy - it is the energy of life itself, it is the energy you are made of. So, check this out: here you are, this infinite energy based being and you keep trying to force yourself to make finite tasks & money more important than love or your health. That is a huge conflict and to stay unaware of it keeps you suffering with health problems (and love & money problems.)

For example, have you ever been guilty of saying anything like the following statements?

"I promise I'll eat better next week."

"After I get these emails written, clean out all of the closets, and reframe the family photos, then I can go to the gym."

"I don't deserve to go to bed yet, I haven't gotten enough work done today."

You've got to be willing to ask yourself, "What would good health do?" in every situation pertaining to your body and health. Sure, you have responsibilities that are important. But, if you are in the habit of neglecting your body's needs and sacrificing your well-being – you SERIOUSLY need to Supercharge Your Health Vibe before you wear your body out! Stay on this training course, please.

So, how do you create a healthy relationship with your body when you are constantly ignoring it, wasting your time doing everything else before taking care of it, and putting what you need to be doing to heal last on the list?

Admitting the problem is always the first step to healing. Use this training course to help you break free of painful habits that hold you back, increase your ability to love your body, and find new ways to unleash the health that is lying dormant inside of you.

Next up: Where's your health mind at and what can you do about it?

CHAPTER 2 - REDEFINE YOUR HEALTH MIND

I hope you already got something helpful from Training Exercise 1. Normally I'm giving this workshop to a group of women at a time, and by this point I've already gotten great feedback that shifts are happening! It's all a part of my master plan to make it as easy as possible for women to feel happy, succeed, and thrive!

But remember,

YOU HAVE TO FULLY PARTICIPATE IN WRITING FOR THIS TO WORK.

Training Exercise 2-1

Without taking a moment to think fill in the blanks with your knee jerk response.

1.   People are _____.

2.   Chocolate is _____.

3.   Music is _____.

4.   Driving is _____.

5.   Traveling is _____.

6.   The Beach is _____.

7.   My body is _____.

8.   Being healthy is _____.

Were your last two answers surprising? I'm going to give you more of a chance to expand on those last two answers because this is the deal; any positive beliefs you have about your body can help you heal and any negative beliefs you have about your body can block health from flowing through you. So let's go on a belief-busting brainstorm.

Training Exercise 2-2

Set a timer for two minutes and write down every negative belief you can find in your mind about health, weakness, recovery, your body, & your looks.

For example: "I never have enough energy to have fun." Ready set go!

_____

_____

_____

_____

_____

_____

_____

_____

_____

_____

_____

_____

_____

_____

_____

_____

_____

_____

_____

_____

_____

_____

_____

_____

Training Exercise 2-3

Ok, it's two minutes later now and you've emptied your mind of negative beliefs and since nature abhors a vacuum, you've got to fill your mind with positive beliefs right away. So now you are going to write the opposite of every negative belief from the above list and turn it into a positive statement. For example: "I never have enough energy to have fun." Becomes, "I have lots of energy to have fun!" Take all take all of the time you need to do this exercise.

_____

_____

_____

_____

_____

_____

_____

_____

_____

_____

_____

_____

_____

_____

_____

_____

_____

_____

_____

_____

_____

MAKE YOUR POSITIVE AFFIRMATIONS

AS POWERFUL AS POSSIBLE:

• Always keep them in present tense.

• Have fun with them.

• Always say them out loud.

• Repeat them often, hundreds of times a day if you can.

• Make sure when you say them you get
some kind of physical sensation in your body.

• Make sure when you say them you get an increase
in emotional feelings.

(Those last 2 are how you know they are working.)

Training Exercise 2-4

Now, read your positive statements out loud. How does it feel when you say those positive statements? Does it feel weird or like a lie? If so, that shows you how strong your negative beliefs are and how hard they are working to block health from easily flowing through you.

There is a lot of misinformation out there about positive affirmations. For one, positive affirmations are not simply thinking positively. They work on deeper physical and consciousness levels than just the realm of thoughts. In fact, scientific studies have concluded that your actual DNA can be changed by both positive and negative thoughts, and that unhealthy cells can be made healthy by deep meditation and the frequency change in your brain that positive thoughts stimulate.[56] In addition to your eye color, you may have also inherited emotional traits through your genes. That's how strong your beliefs are![7]

Here are my 6 points of clarity
about positive affirmations from an energetic perspective.

1. **If your beliefs aren't working for you they are working against you.** Some of your beliefs are life supporting, some bring you down. The ones that bring you down THINK THEY ARE PROTECTING you, THEY THINK THEY ARE LIFE SUPPORTING beliefs – but they are wrong. When you identify the beliefs that bring you down, it feels weird and scary to try to change them. But if they are not working for you, they are working against you – and that makes life hard and good health scarce.

2. **You are always creating from both your conscious and unconscious mind.** That is why it is so important to change those bummer beliefs, so you can consciously create a life you want instead of feeling like a victim of a life you don't like so much. Form follows thought. So you want to make sure that your thoughts are headed in the direction you want your life to go.

3. **Ultimate health is an open flow of energy.** Control is a tight squeezing energy. So it isn't that positive affirmations give you control, it's that they give the energy of your thoughts a direction. Constantly directing energy towards your vision of a happy healthy life gives you a better chance of having one.

4. **Thoughts get stuck in habitual loops in the brain.**[8] A positive affirmation changes course by making a whole new neural pathway!   This is incredible! As you learned if you ever heard my live presentation, there is now

scientific proof that you can actually re-wire and new wire your physical brain. That takes 30-40 days of consistent new thoughts, talk, and behavior.[9] So let's get you on the path of creating new healthy habits in your brain today.

5.   **Like attracts like.** The positive affirmation is like a magnet, and it makes your energy field change vibrational frequencies from what you don't want to what you do want, and that magnetically attracts like energy to you. If you are radiating at a dis-eased frequency, you attract more dis-ease. Feel like a loser, you lose. Worry about not having a healthy body, you don't. Radiate at healthy frequencies and you attract better life situations and a healthier body. Keep reading and practicing and you will succeed at doing this!

6.   **Just be willing.** If the positive statement feels just too far fetched, you can back it up a bit until you can feel more of a vibrational match with it. For example, if, "Love always heals" is too much of a stretch for you, try this instead, "I am willing for love to always heal." That opens up your energy flow, and open energy flow is what transformation is all about!

While I provide plenty of scientific studies to back all of this up, the most direct proof is in how you feel after the positive affirmations help get you over the resistance phase. I have been working with this within my own mind and supporting clients in doing the same for decades, and the results in how much better each of us feels is astounding. When I think scary, sad, hopeless thoughts, I feel scared, sad, and hopeless. When I think fun, happy, positive thoughts, I get to feel happy and excited about life. I get more creative and feel energized when I direct my thoughts towards what I do want to experience instead of obsessing about my fears.

You want to feel better? Think better thoughts.

It's worked for me and millions of others. You just have to stick to it for at least a month for it to really start to take hold, get easier, and gain momentum. Then the positive thoughts start to automatically replace the negative thoughts. In the very least, it results in you feeling better. At the best, you create enjoyable new life experiences. That alone seems worth sticking with this training.

So far you've gotten clear on what you want good health for, you've emptied out your negative health and body beliefs and replaced them with positive ones, you've gotten the lowdown on why positive affirmations are so powerful, and you know how you can use them every day to become a good health and vitality magnet. Repeat your positive statements out loud every day and let this sink in and start making new healthy neural pathways in your brain as you also supercharge your health vibration in your energy system. Then you'll be ready to go to the next level in Supercharging Your Health Vibe!

> "We are what we repeatedly do;
> excellence then is not an act, but a habit."
> - Aristotle

Next up: Neediness & Worthiness.

CHAPTER 3 - NEEDY BY NATURE WORTHY BY EXISTENCE

This next topic comes up a lot with my clients and it was something that I had to heal to supercharge my health vibe. Let me ask you this: If all humans are indeed created equal, is it true that you could be "less than" any other human on the planet?

No. No possible way.

Yet so many people have issues around placing themselves below another person. And that gets tied in with neediness and feeling guilty for having any kind of need… at all… ever.

I could go on and on about self worth and neediness, it's long and convoluted and full of psychological gymnastics. But I'm here to help you heal, so I like to keep the healing effective and results oriented, so I come back to two basic facts:

1.   We are all created equal, so I can't be better or worse or deserve more or less than anyone else.

2.   We are human, therefore, we have needs.

You have basic survival needs: air, food, water, shelter. Then you have basic thrive needs such as: respect, understanding, trust, love. (For a complete list of Basic Human Needs please refer to Rosenberg, Marshal B. (2003) "Non-Violent

Communication: A Language of Life" and Maslow, A.H. (1943). "A theory of human motivation." *Psychological Review* 50 (4) 370–96.)

When you were born, you needed constant care from others or you would have died. You were totally dependent. As you grew, you gradually learned to take care of your own needs and become more independent. As you matured, you learned when it's best to take care of yourself and when it's best to ask for help. Well, in a perfect world you learned when it's best to take care of yourself and when it's best to ask for help, but you may really struggle with asking for help or taking care of yourself first.

Can you relate to this? You vacillate between feeling helpless and co-dependent, thinking lowly of yourself, and devaluing your skills - to taking every burden onto your shoulders and striking out alone, doing it all yourself and not accepting/asking for help. I've noticed after more than 2 decades of helping people heal that a lot of suffering occurs by vacillating between these two painful places.

> The truth remains, you are human therefore you have needs, so you've got to accept the fact that you are needy by nature and worthy by existence and let that set you free.

When you fight against your healthy, natural human needs you create an energy block in your system that keeps you from receiving the love, health, and money you want. You deny the basic natural order that all beings are created equal when you put yourself down, hold yourself back, and think negative thoughts about yourself or your body.

Whenever you take on too much by yourself without receiving help when you really could use it, you tell the Universe that you DON'T want the gifts it has for you. The Universe sent you a person or thing to help you out, and you told the Universe "NO." So then the Universe gets the message, "Oh, she can't receive so she obviously doesn't want to be given nice things. Ok, got it. Don't give her nice things."

Conversely, when you don't stand strongly on your own two feet, and strike out on your own sometimes, you deny the magnificently resilient energy you are made of the chance to prove to you your inner strength.

It might seem tricky, but you can learn how to be strong on your own -AND- strong asking for help. Your words, thoughts, feelings, and actions are training the Universe – and other people - how to treat you. If you want to receive better health, you must allow yourself to be honest about your true worth and your true needs as they truly are in each moment. That's a lot of truthiness.

Sometimes what blocks your ability to supercharge your health vibe is feelings of guilt from someone you've wronged in the past, so you feel like you don't deserve to feel good. You may have hurt yourself or someone else so deeply that you can't forgive yourself.

Here is my recipe for forgiveness:

1) Apologize to the person/people you hurt. Take responsibility WITHOUT EXCUSES for the painful action and sincerely say, "I'm sorry I did _____. I feel true remorse. I know it was painful and I sincerely apologize. I am truly sorry.

2) Ask what you can do to make amends, then actually follow through and do it. Even if you can't actually make up for it, you can still take action to help the healing process. Yes, you can even do this for yourself when you've hurt yourself!

3) Become trustworthy by taking whatever healthy action you can to improve your behavior and promise YOURSELF that you will not do the harmful action again.

4) If you knew better you would do better, and now you know better. But at the time you did the harmful thing, you might have been doing the best you could for the awareness you had. Accept that you are human and make mistakes, and be willing to forgive yourself. Forgiveness can be hard to do and you can't force true forgiveness. So, just be willing to forgive yourself.

5) The other person may or may not be able to forgive you and that is their right. Apologize, take responsibility for your part, make amends through positive action, be willing to forgive yourself, and let the other person have their feelings about you, no matter what they are. Give them the freedom they deserve because...

> "Would you rather be right or free?"
> ~ Byron Katie

I choose love and freedom and hope you can too.

Training Exercise 3-1

Remember, at your core you are not better or worse than anyone else, and they are not better or worse than you. You are equal and no more or less deserving.

Without comparing yourself to anyone else, write down 3 skills you have that you enjoy.

1. _____
2. _____
3. _____

Next to each skill write how that benefits your life.

For example:

a)   Skill I enjoy: Making costumes.

Benefit to self: Fun, move creative energy, joy, problem solving, communion with Dale (my man.)

b)   Skill I enjoy: Seeing both sides of an argument.

Benefit to self: Feel love and equanimity, exercise my brain, grow my capacity to love and accept, communion with fellow humans.

c)   Skill I enjoy: Hiking.

Benefit to self: Ground, improve coordination & fitness, connect with nature, see new things from a new perspective.

Now it's your turn:

1.   Skill I enjoy:_____

How I benefit:_____

2.   Skill I enjoy:_____

How I benefit:_____

3.   Skill I enjoy:_____

How I benefit:_____

Great, write all of that down for real. This course will not supercharge your health vibe if you do it all in your head. You MUST bring it into the physical realm by writing it down.

Next to your above written answers, fill in how that might benefit others.

For example:

1.   Making costumes.

Benefit to self: Fun, move creative energy, joy, problem solving, communion with Dale

Benefit to others: people laugh, feel inspired, and lighten up. Move creative energy on the planet.

2.   Seeing both sides of an argument.

Benefit to self: Feel love and equanimity, exercise my brain, grow my capacity to love and accept, communion with fellow humans.

Benefit to others: Increase love and respect between humans on the planet, decrease war promote peace.

3.   Hiking.

Benefit to self: Grounding, Improve coordination & fitness, connect with nature.

Benefit to others: I often help people with directions when I hike, inspire others to get fit, I clean up trails, I give money to the Sierra club and to support national and state parks that protect land, I give money to manufacturers of quality gear, I increase respect for mother earth and keep healthy energy moving on the planet, I take women hiking with me the first Saturday of every month.

1. Skill I enjoy:_____

How I benefit:_____

How another benefits:_____

2. Skill I enjoy:_____

How I benefit:_____

How another benefits:_____

3.Skill I enjoy:_____

How I benefit:_____

How another benefits:_____

See? Just doing the things you enjoy doing

can be a benefit to others!

Now sit back and bask in the glow

of what a valuable asset you are!

Training Exercise 3-2

Do you ever find yourself saying really mean things inside your own head? Well guess what? Self-deprecating talk won't get you better health. That mean trash talk will only hold you back as your loveless words deny the power that is the wondrous energy you are made of. Honoring the truth of your very Being is what opens up the good health super highway because it supercharges the energy frequency you're putting out to the world, which affects what you get back from the world. So start shifting this right here right now.

Stand up.

Get up off of your butt.

Shake it out then plant your feet shoulder width apart.

Say out loud…

"I love myself as I am.

I am worthy of great health.

I am worthy of peace.

I am worthy of healthy whole food.

I allow all of the vibrant health I want to easily come to me and

I receive it.

I feel healthiness all around me.

I take fantastic care of myself."

Niiiice. Try saying this before every meal for the next week. No, I'm not kidding. Write it down on several post-its. Place it in the center of your steering wheel, on your mirror, in your pocket, & in your wallet!   Repeat it as often as you possible, hundreds of times a day! You want to make a strong neural pathway of self worth so that you can supercharge your health vibe.

Training Exercise 3-3
Go from mean trash talk – to Luscious Love Lips for the next 24 hours!

There is an old saying I learned from Florence Scovel Shinn that reminds you of the power of your words: "YOUR WORD IS YOUR WAND." Every time you hear yourself say, or about to say, something like, "I'm so scared I'll always be sick." Use your word as your wand to state what you DO want instead. "I'm so happy that my body heals more every day!" "I'm so relieved that at least half of my plate was vegetables at all 3 meals today." – you can say that on your way to lunch, imprint what you do what to happen onto your subconscious mind. Have fun with it. Some of my favorite mantras, "I take care of myself and get enough sleep tonight." "I find something to love about my body every day!" "I love and accept myself as I am." Now that's luscious love lips!

Try this for 24 hours, no mean trash talk, only words of love – then see how you feel. If you say mean trash talk within the 24 hour time frame, the count starts over from hour 1 again.
The more you do it, the stronger you feel and the easier it gets! I guarantee that will supercharge your health vibe and you will want to keep it up.

If you have deep issues around self worth, guilt, needs, and deserving, don't worry, you really can heal these issues and come to a whole new way of being and feeling in your life. Keep moving forward through this training course, and if you'd like more help on your healing journey, I'm here for you.

Next up: Make your peace with the natural flow of the Universe.

CHAPTER 4 - THE NATURAL FLOW OF THE UNIVERSE: GIVING AND RECEIVING

Now that you own that you are a worthy human being, you accept that you are a human therefor you have needs, and you reprogrammed your system to allow health to come to you, let's get you in harmony with the most natural cycle in life: Giving and Receiving.

A carrot plant receives sunshine, rain, and nutrients from the soil so it can grow, it then gives us nutrients for our health, we exhale and the carrot plant receives our carbon dioxide giving us back oxygen.

> Giving and receiving is how life on earth is sustained.

But if you've been traumatized, verbally or physically abused, or just were somehow given confusing messages about safety, food, or nurturance, it's really hard to simply receive because what came to you in the past wasn't always safe, wanted, or right for your wellbeing.

The problem now is that by trying to protect yourself from harmful things, you also block the flow of good things coming to you! Giving and receiving are a two way street on one road that needs to keep clear so the flow can go back and forth in a natural harmonious way.

> You can't change the past, but you can decide to open yourself to the goodness the Universe has for you today.

Training Exercise 4-1

1.   Place your hands on a part of your body that could use some extra healing. Healing happens in connection, and usually if something is hurting or sick, we tend to disconnect or pull away from it, while simultaneously dwelling on it in our mind. It's a weird ignore/obsess cycle that blocks healing. Think of how gently you touch a baby, or a puppy, or hug your mom – so much love gets conveyed in that touch. Touch your own body in that gentle and loving way.

2.   Take 3 breaths in and out of this area where your hands are placed.

3.   Very gently, and with love in your voice, speak to this area of your body, "I am open to receive great health and I safely receive it now. I allow the health inside me to grow. I envision my body fully healed."

4.   Allow yourself to actually see yourself fully healed. What might you do differently if you were 100% healthy? Imagine yourself doing that for the next few minutes.

5.   Do this exercise as many times as you like with every part of your body that you judge or that is sick or injured. You will start to see a difference in not only how you feel, but also how you think about and relate with your body.

Training Exercise 4-2

When you think about something, your brain thinks it is actually happening.[10] [11] So, give yourself permission anywhere, anytime, to think about the abundance of health and vitality that is all around you. When you notice plentiful things, it rings an abundance bell in your personal energy field, and you want to ring that abundance bell a lot to help supercharge your health vibe. Remember the tuning forks? This exercise works like that![12]

All I have to do is think about it and I can feel myself hiking up Mount Hollywood in the spring. The wildflowers are bursting out everywhere and the air smells fresh! I think about kittens playing and rolling around so cute and full of life and I can imagine what that must feel like. I recall the Aspen trees in the Rocky Mountains; row after row, their roots all connected under the earth. I remember looking up at the Milky Way, billions of stars sparkling in the sky. Those things get me right into feeling the abundant vitality of the Universe, and my whole being vibrates with that abundant well-being. I can take it even further and imagine myself doing things that seem difficult. Like I imagined myself climbing up 75 flights of stairs in the tallest building West of the Mississippi for years before I got up the nerve to tackle it for a local charity. Now it is a yearly event for the Happy Woman Academy and I look forward to it with enjoyment!

There is a huge difference in your vibration when you allow yourself to have what you want, if only in your thoughts and feelings, because it sets up a positive condition to allow you to get what you want in your body. Get it? And depending on the severity of your medical condition, sometimes your imagination is the best thing you've got. So let it run wild and enjoy thinking about fun things you'd like to do and really feel yourself doing it, instead of thinking about not being able to do it, totally go for it in your mind. Especially if imagination is all you've got because of low physical function, it will supercharge your health vibe to enjoy imagining that you are actually doing the fun things you'd like to do, whether or not you can actually ever do them.

Around Christmas of 1989 I was so sick with Hepatitis A that I couldn't move and was only awake for 1 hour per day. I felt horribly lonely because I was in quarantine. My mind was perfectly sharp, but my body could barely function and I felt imprisoned inside my body. I didn't know if I would recover and I felt very scared.

One of the only things that helped me at that time was thinking about Nelson Mandela, who had been in prison for 27 years. He was released on Feb 11th, 1990, while I was still very weak, and I heard him say, "As I walked out the door toward the gate that would lead to my freedom, I knew if I didn't leave my bitterness and hatred behind, I'd still be in prison." When that bitterness and hatred is in your mind, it poisons your body and makes you feel even worse than your illness does. I decided I was going to focus on whatever shred of positivity and good feeling I could muster up. Three days later I was feeling stronger and out of quarantine and I was able to fly to visit my family on the South East Coast. Amazing!

I know it is challenging, but please, give yourself the chance to supercharge your health vibe by practicing all I teach here and by imagining yourself well. It really will help you to feel better.

Next, let's clear up a common misconception around giving and receiving. People often have negative ideas that giving means: giving it all away, overdoing it from obligation, or giving yourself up. They also have negative ideas that receiving means: taking or being selfish - and those negative ideas make guilt and shame grow. Those concepts are the dark side of giving and receiving that get expressed when you are out of balance, but there is a light side too! When you are in touch with your loving heart and living in balance, you give and receive equally, happily, and cleanly. This is the way that both giving and receiving feel awesome.

If you try to separate giving from receiving you'll feel exhausted, overwhelmed, resentful, get sick easily, and your health problems will persist. It's necessary to receive rest, love, healthy food, money, & joy, so that you can give it back to your body and to other people.

I've made it my life's mission to help women keep their successful [13]career without sacrificing their health or relationships. If you rob energy from your health, children, or marriage in order to keep your career going – you will crash and burn and end up sabotaging all you hold dear. Every aspect of your life will suffer if you don't put your well-being at the top of your list. You can't give from a dry well forever and all of that giving from obligation makes you resentful as well as depleted and exhausted. I've seen it too many times in my clients and I witnessed it in my mother and grandmother who neglected their own well-being and marriages in the name of work and the glorification of busy. Tending to your inner world is serious business. I'm so glad you are committed to seeing this training course all of the way through so that you can give and receive in just the right amount to keep you healthy, wealthy, and in love with your life.

So let's continue to unstick the places you might be stuck and open up the giving and the receiving flow of energy inside of you, bringing your inner and outer world into harmony and supercharging your health vibe.

Training Exercise 4-3

Stand up.

Get out of your chair and move.

Shake your body, shake it out.

If you can't physically get up that's ok, just do the best you can from the position you are in.

Plant your feet shoulder width apart, bend your knees, and place both hands on the center of your breastbone over your heart energy center. Now think of one of your closest friends. Think of how much goodness you want this person to have. Doesn't it feel great to love them and wish them good things?

See your friend in your mind's eye and imagine giving your friend a big hug. Shine out your love to them. See them happy and smiling and healthy. Imagine them safe and having what they want and need to feel good. Remember a time when you laughed so hard together that you had no thoughts, just pure joy running through you. Go ahead, send your dear friend a big blast of love from your heart.

Yes, that feels so great to give your love, care, and positive thoughts to this wonderful loving person. Take some moments and do not move on to the next section until you stand up, plant your feet should width apart, and actually do this exercise right now. Aaaah… that feels amazing!

Take a deep cleansing breath.

Training Exercise 4-4

Now let yourself remember the kind things this person has done for you. Think about the times they had your back, cheered you up, celebrated with you, and supported you. Take a deep breath into your heart, fling your arms wide open, and shout out loud,

"THANK YOU FOR LOVING ME!"

You've got to let yourself actually physically and verbally do this. (Or you can just keep blocking the good health you say you want.)   You can do it!   Prove to the Universe you are ready to receive. Really feel the gratitude you have for your friend's love and care. Let their love in. Soak up their love and care like a giant sea sponge of love. Allow their wonderful giving to shower you and sink into you. (This exercise always makes me tear up. I just did it again while reading over this exercise, my eyes are leaking.)

It feels so great when I give to someone and they sincerely appreciate it. But, giving doesn't feel as good when the other person does not happily receive it. I want to see the people I love happy. I know you want to let yourself receive because you are taking this training course. You will automatically supercharge your health vibe as you supercharge your ability to receive. So, allow yourself to truly receive when people do nice things for you, then your receiving becomes the gift you give back to them.

That is how it works here on earth. Do you want to receive more? You have to make sure you are OPEN and that your giving comes from your loving heart and that you let yourself receive with joy and gratitude.

Try doing these two Training Exercises with at least 2 more people in mind. Get very specific about seeing your loved ones in your mind's eye and giving then receive a big love blast to and from them.

I understand that it can seem scary or hard to receive, that is why I want you to practice by thinking of people that you trust and love, so that your energy system can learn what it feels like to safely receive, heal, and get better and better at receiving. As you practice doing it in the safety and privacy of your own space alone, you'll build strength to be able to do it with people and things outside of your little world. Keep going, you are doing great!

Next up: A way to practice gratitude that really works to supercharge your health vibe.

CHAPTER 5 - SHOW GRATITUDE IN WHAT YOU THINK, SAY, AND DO!

It's important to practice strengthening the energy frequency of gratitude in regards to health because gratitude tells the Universe, "Yes please. Give me more of this good stuff I like. Thank you!" I mean hey, when someone sincerely says, "Thank you" to you, doesn't it automatically make you want to give them more? Yes! See, the Universe works just like you do!

Pain, disease, and lack of fitness can bring attention to what you don't like about your body. But have you ever stopped to think about everything going RIGHT in your body right now? Do you know how many processes are happening as you sit there reading?

Let's see, there are 11 entire systems that run a human body and they are all functioning and interacting at some level of success right now because you are alive. When you consider that in this moment your body is: bending light so you can read these words, extracting nutrients from food, producing lymphatic fluid, equalizing body temperature, producing hormones, removing carbon dioxide, creating neuropeptides, pumping blood, nourishing tissue, lifting your hand to turn the page, shifting so you can be more comfortable, and your skin is keeping it all in – it is pretty astounding! Every one of those actions involves more muscles, fluid, bacteria, and nerve activity than you could imagine. Your heart beat 72 times and your blood traveled 117,000 miles in just the last minute![14]

Without you even realizing it, your body is doing all it can to achieve homeostasis right now. Homeostasis is a healthy balance of chemicals & processes that keep a body optimally functioning. Your body is trying hard to keep you healthy right now. Isn't that something worth feeling extremely grateful about?

Training Exercise 5-1

What about your body has you feeling angry or sad? Don't keep it bottled up inside, go ahead and let it out. Let that pain flow out of your body, through the pen, onto the page.

_____

_____

_____

_____

_____

_____

_____

_____

_____

_____

_____

_____

Good. It's important to be honest about your emotions, feel them, and let them flow through you. You don't need to hurt yourself with your emotions; you just need to feel them. You don't need to hurt anyone else with your emotions; you just need to feel them. There is nothing bad or wrong about uncomfortable emotions, allow them to move through you completely without harming yourself or anyone else.

Uncomfortable emotions are not the problem. Staying stuck in them for too long is where you get into trouble. If you feel sad, go ahead and have a good cry.

If you feel angry, anger moves better with physical action, but if you are too sick or injured to move, the anger can get bottled up inside of you. So, you have to imagine that you are running hard, boxing it out, or doing Kung Fu. In fact, in your imagination you can do some things that maybe you wouldn't dare do in real life, even if you could! So only if you can't physically exert yourself to move anger through you do you get a free pass to imagine it. Otherwise, you've got to physically move it move it! Run, exercise hard, punch a pile of pillows, punch a punching bag with gloves & your wrists wrapped, go to kick boxing class… whatever you can do that physically allows you to kick and punch and burn through the anger SAFELY without harming yourself or another. If you've bottled up anger for a long time and expressing it is totally new for you, I strongly suggest you find a Core Energetics Therapist to help you. https://www.coreenergetics.org/

All emotions are Energy in MOTION –

and emotions are made to move.

Training Exercise 5-2

Circle the answers that are truest for you:

1. Which way would you rather feel?
   o   Angry and Sad
   o   Accepting and Grateful

2. Which vibrations do you think are more likely to attract the health you want?
   o   Angry and Sad
   o   Accepting and Grateful

3. When you take stock, do you think it is fair to say that your body is doing more correctly in this moment than you had previously thought?
   o   Yes
   o   No

4. Are you more likely to want to help someone if they psupercharge you or criticize you?
   o   Psupercharge
   o   Criticize

5. Is it time to be more thankful for everything your body is doing right in every single moment, rather than to put it down for the things it is doing that you don't like?
   o   Yes
   o   No

6. Learning what you have so far from this book, do you think it is possible that your body would like hearing you psupercharge and give thanks to it more than hearing you criticize it?

o Yes

o No

7. If it was scientifically proven that speaking, thinking, and acting kindly to your body could improve your health, would you do it?

o Yes

o No

Believe it or not, molecular biologists have proven that your genes get manipulated by how your mind perceives and interprets your environment. A positive or a negative attitude sends messages to the cells in your body and can actually reprogram their health and behavior. It can even change DNA and cellular structure; repairing diseased cells.[15] You might want to read those sentences a few more times and let them sink in. You have more power to heal than you thought.

A lot of people think acceptance is the same as submission or giving up. But I feel a different vibration from the word acceptance. To me, acceptance means stating "what is" in the present moment and keeping the door open for it to change. When you try to control something, it has a tight squeezing effect on your energy channels. Like when you are tense and your muscles tighten up.

Stress, worrying, blaming, and fighting, "what is" also squeeze your energy channels. But in order to be healthy, energy needs to flow on open channels. When there is a kink in the hose, the energy can't flow to make you healthier. ACCEPTING what is happening in the moment and simultaneously staying open to it changing allows vital energy to move through you.

Training Exercise 5-3

Write down 5 things about your body that you are very grateful for.

For example: I'm so grateful that my heart is beating right now!

1. _____
2. _____
3. _____
4. _____
5. _____

Training Exercise 5-4

Write down 5 NEW thoughts you could think that would show more gratitude and appreciation towards your body. Even if you are sick or hurting, find a way to think with thanks. For example if you have any sickness right now: "Thank you lymphatic fluid for doing your best to make me healthy. I really appreciate how hard you are working to heal me." (Do you think your body might like hearing that better than, "Stupid body. Why are you still sick?")

Ok, it is your turn, you can do this!

1. _____
2. _____
3. _____
4. _____
5. _____

Don't you wish you were appreciated more? So does your body! Give it the appreciation and gratitude that it truly deserves. Go ahead, take a deep breath, place both hands over your heart chakra in the middle of your breastbone, and sincerely thank your body for supporting you. An attitude of gratitude and saying THANK YOU when people & things add goodness to your life strengthens your health vibe.

Training Exercise 5-5

Write down 5 ways that you could have a dialogue between your body and yourself. Then say "thank you" every day in a kind way that you know your body would like to hear. For example:

"Thanks Elizabeth for remembering to stretch after hiking today."

"Sure thing body! Thanks for getting me up that mountain with gusto! That was fun!"

Ok, you might feel silly doing this, but it actually works to move energy and supercharge your health vibe!

1._____

_____

2._____

_____

3._____

_____

4. _____

_____

5. _____

_____

Training Exercise 5-6

Write down 5 actions you can take that express love and gratitude to your body in a way that you know it will like.

For example: Take an Epsom salt bath every night. Put on music in the morning and dance while making breakfast. Go to spin class. (I've done these things this weekend. I really want my body to know how much I love it and how grateful I am for it!)

1._____

2._____

3._____

4. _____

5._____

Then take action and do at least one nurturing thing for your body every day until you die. Keep coming up with new ways to show your love and appreciation for your awesome body!   Good health is like a campfire. You don't just light it once and expect it to keep burning. You have to tend to the fire every few minutes, putting in new kindling, nudging logs around, throwing a new log on the fire. That is the only way the fire keeps burning and that is the only way your body stays healthy! And instead of being tiring, it is actually energizing and it picks up momentum and gets easier to do.

Training Exercise 5-7

Think back to a time when something happened that you did NOT want to happen, yet, somehow something EVEN BETTER happened because of it. Write about what you learned from that experience, and the GOOD that came from it. (PS: this is a VERY important training exercise, no skipping over it.)

_____

_____

_____

_____

_____

_____

_____

_____

_____

_____

_____

_____

_____

_____

_____

_____

_____

_____

_____

_____

_____

_____

_____

_____

See, sometimes you think things are going wrong, when actually they are going right! This training exercise proves how important it is to be as thankful as possible in your thoughts, words, and actions every day, no matter what is happening in your life.

I'm always amazed by people with chronic or deadly illness or who have survived horrific accidents and are maimed, yet they still have a positive attitude. I've been sick for months at a time, been badly injured and have done years of rehab, I've had 9 concussions, many broken bones, and several surgeries, and I was usually pretty cranky about it. It was been difficult for me to find a silver lining at the time. But somehow, many people can do it and I find them incredibly inspirational! I've been working on supercharging my health vibe for a long time, and I'm getting much better at finding something positive about the painful things I've been through. If people that have been hurt much worse than I have are able to find something positive in their challenging situation, than I can as well and so can you.

Training Exercise 5-8

If you are or have been sick or injured, try to find something to be grateful for that has come from it. Do at least 2 now, but keep this exercise going and list as many as you can over time. Let's join forces and supercharge this part of our health vibe together! I'll go first:

1. The last 2 times I required foot surgery, I found an incredible surgeon who is also an incredibly cool human. He allowed me to not only stay awake during surgery and watch, but with his staff's assistance I held a live Facebook event with my iPhone! My friends and I posted back and forth and I posted photos in real time throughout the procedure. It was empowering! I feel incredibly grateful for a positive surgery experience and the excellent Dr. Sadrieh at Evo Foot Clinic.

2. Even though I eat healthily and am fit, I got gallbladder disease 3 years ago and

it was horribly painful. I didn't want to have my gallbladder removed, and with the help of a dear friend, I found the most amazing Acupuncturist who used to be an M.D. who helped me heal without resorting to surgery. She is my go to doctor for every sniffle and problem now, and I've sent nearly all of my friends and LA clients to her. She's a Godsend, and I never would have found her unless I got that desperate because acupuncture had never helped me much in the past. Also, Dr. Tsoy's special herbs cleared up adult cystic acne that I had for 30 years and had spent $60k on trying to heal. Incredibly grateful to have her in my life!

Now it's your turn:

1. _____

_____

_____

_____

_____

_____

_____

_____

2. _____

_____

_____

_____

_____

_____

_____

_____

Remember, you work how the Universe works – the Universe works how you work. You love being thanked and it makes you want to give more. The Universe loves being thanked and it makes it want to give you more. Your body loves being thanked and it makes you want to heal more! Test drive this law of universal energy flow. I've been using it for years to feel healthier and I am living proof that the exercises in this book work!

In fact, listen to this story. I have the kind of vertigo that is caused by the tiny bones of the inner ear taking a wander and hitting up against the balance center, which makes me feel like I'm on the ocean in a small boat in a raging storm. A few weeks ago I went to sleep feeling happy and whole on a Saturday night, and awoke Sunday morning dizzy and totally nauseated. As horribly sick as I felt, I just kept thanking my body for taking care of me and doing the best it could. I made a nest of pillows and blankets on the bathroom floor, and laid there writhing in headache pain and occasionally vomiting while the room spun around me. BUT my mood never dropped. I used the 5 steps over and over that I teach in my "Happy Woman Formula" as well as exercises that I teach you in this book. I knew that the exercises worked, but that was really a trial by fire! After 2 hours of intense pain I realized that I couldn't take it any more. I closed my eyes and decided I was ready to die. I silently said goodbye to my loved ones, laid back onto the pillows, and passed out cold.

A couple of hours later I awoke and the extreme nausea was gone, but the head pain and spinning was still present – and I thanked and thanked my body for all of the good work it had done while I slept. Of course I had to cancel my work for that day, yet despite the pain, I felt calm, happy, and at peace. It was a good day.

Infusing your thoughts, words, feelings and actions with an extra dose of gratitude gives you the power to create your own healthy vibrant world. That is what practicing these training exercises has done for me, and that is what they can do for you.

Next up: Why wait to feel the health you want?

CHAPTER 6 - DON'T WAIT, FEEL HEALTHY NOW!

So, you know why you want to supercharge your health vibe, but don't you also wonder what it would FEEL like to have so much overflowing health that you feel it all of the time – even when you are sick or injured? Sure that might sound contradictory, but I can do it so I know you can too. Get out ahead of the physical world manifestation and start feeling better in every way that you can. The truth is, you don't have to wait for all of your health problems to be resolved in order for you to feel good. You can start small by doing little things that make you feel healthy without waiting for outside circumstances to change. And that sure beats feeling miserable on top of pain.

Training Exercise 6-1

Write down 3 ways you can boost your healthy feelings.

For example:

1. I can dance around the house more often.

2. I can take my vitamins after each meal.

3. I can imagine my body feels happy as I hike the West Highland Way!

1. _____

2. _____

3. _____

Training Exercise 6-2

There is a vibrant healthy person inside of you just waiting to be unleashed! Take 3 super slow and deep breaths while you allow the health you already have inside of you to come alive and on the fourth breath say out loud,

"I activate the good health within me. I feel healthy now!"

Training Exercise 6-3

Write down 3 ways that you already feel healthy in your life.

1. _____

2. _____

3. _____

Over the next few weeks, keep noticing ways that you already feel healthy and really let yourself enjoy feeling it each time. This strengthens your good health muscles and supercharges your health vibe.

The inner secret to shift from dis-ease to health is always about imagining it, saying it, feeling it, and letting your actions and the actions of the Universe respond to your vibrations. Like sonar waves emanating out from you, your vibration both attracts and repels. So you want to be sending out the right vibes that attract what you DO want to happen in your life. New thoughts appear, new circumstances arise, and new actions get taken when you change your thoughts and your energy from focusing on what is wrong to focusing on the true abundance of the energy you are made of and resonating with the good health within and around you.

Feeling energized, happy, and vital are a part of what you want good health for anyway - so why wait until you have absolutely no aches, pains, or issues? Give yourself those feelings now and cut a clear pathway that allows good health to easily flow through you, and then you can Feel healthy and BE healthy in this moment. Not some potential future date, but right NOW. Feel everything you want right now

"I Am Totally Healthy and Thriving NOW."

If you keep thinking and talking about the gap from where you are to where you want to be – guess what happens? That gap widens!! You have the power to eradicate that gap. Feel what you want to feel NOW; don't wait for some imaginary future.

Today I finally find myself with the man of my dreams after decades of abusive relationships. He is intelligent, funny, sexy, so caring, and we have very similar values. How did he find me? Every morning I wouldn't let myself get out of bed until I had a genuine smile on my face and FELT what it would feel like to be in the perfect relationship for me. After 6 months of doing this every morning before I got up and every night before I went to sleep, the comments started: "Have you met someone?"

"You look like you're in love." "You are glowing." "Are you in love?" I would always answer the same way, "I'm in love, I just haven't met him yet!" But you know what, I had that tickly "in love feeling" inside All Day Every Day. I no longer pined, I no longer lamented, I was in LOVE!

I kept radiating that love vibe exactly how I wanted it to be and my sonar waves attracted my man to me like a magnet. So don't deny that everything isn't already inside of you. Keep practicing and let yourself feel healthy, and anything else you want to feel, NOW.

You can start small by doing little things that make you feel healthy without exerting yourself. If you want to get fit, but just can't seem to make it to a gym regularly, get a buddy to take walks or go dance with. It is always easier when you have an accountability partner to get you motivated and keep you on track. That worked for me after 42 years of inconsistent exercise. Once a friend committed to going to the gym with me, neither one of us wanted to let the other down! Whatever might be a fun way for you to move your body, maybe even try something new. I am not a sporty person, but I secretly always wanted to play beach volleyball. I didn't even know how to play volleyball or what the rules were, but I joined a Meetup.com group and headed to the beach for 5 hours every Saturday. I stank at volleyball, but I had an absolute blast and got a major workout. Plus, that is where I met my incredible man and we've been together since 2008 and are still going strong!! See, you never know all of the great things a healthy lifestyle can bring to you!

Training Exercise 6-4

a) Tonight, after you get into bed, allow yourself to feel healthy now. Imagine yourself in very specific scenarios. What does it look like around you? What is the temperature? Are you at home? Traveling? Walking down the street? Having dinner with friends? Swimming in the ocean? You can choose a different scene every time if you want. Get creative and let your imagination run wild. Whatever it is you WANT to feel by having the health you desire, that is how you allow yourself to feel, right now, as you lay there falling asleep. Sweet dreams.

b) When you wake up in the morning, allow yourself to have those same healthy feelings RIGHT AWAY. Don't hesitate or else dis-ease can set in quickly and make you feel sick. You are doing this training to supercharge your health vibe, so supercharge it first thing in the morning and keep it going all day – no matter how your body feels, there is still health alive inside of you waiting to be unleashed. Your job is to unleash it! Keep practicing. Your inner health will keep getting magnified and stronger and you'll gain momentum towards feeling better.

So far you've already shifted health beliefs that were holding you back, supercharged your inner health vibration, opened the flow of giving and receiving, gotten clear on what you want health for, shifted to an attitude of gratitude, and started to vibrate at the energetic frequency of health now... But are you in alignment? Find out in chapter lucky #7!

Next Up: Get Into Centered Alignment

CHAPTER 7 - GET INTO CENTERED ALIGNMENT

If you've been putting into practice all that you've learned along this workbook, you've probably already seen some shifts in your physical world and how you feel about your body. By this point Many women have told me little and big things that have healed, which is very exciting. Be sure to read and practice all the way to the end of this book.

Have you ever noticed that sometimes you are just totally in the zone and everything comes easily to you and you are just getting stuff done like a boss? Then there are times where doing even the things you enjoy is like trying to push a boulder up a hill? When I'm struggling against the current, feeling miserable, and putting tons of effort into something but not enjoying it at all because there is no flow, I know what is wrong. I'm out of centered alignment. Centered alignment with what? With my innate power and highest good in that moment.

Allow me to explain.

You may have so many responsibilities and things you "have to get done" that your life is run by all of those obligations and outside forces determining your every move. When you live that way, life feels like a grind. Even simple things like folding laundry or driving to work are a struggle. But when your actions are preceded by aligning with your highest good and bringing yourself to your centered inner power, even doing the dishes can feel joyful, and your meaningful work/ art/ studying/ parenting, FEELS FANTASTIC TO DO!

WHEN YOU ARE IN CENTERED ALIGNMENT WITH YOUR HIGHEST GOOD:

• Creativity is boosted and new ideas keep popping up

• You roll up your sleeves and joyfully take care of business

• Challenges get tackled and feel satisfying

• You enjoy taking care of your body and make sure you get enough exercise, nourishing food, and rest.

• When sudden changes occur you go with the flow and don't let it throw you off.

• You get paid your worth and money flows to you more easily.

• You feel happy about today and excited about your future.

• You feel in love - not just with your partner, but with life.

Do you want to feel that way every day? I do! I teach an immersive program on how to bring yourself into centered alignment with your highest good called the "Happy Woman Formula." Go to www.TheHappyWomanAcademy.com so you can get in on that action – you'll even get to find out the #1 way you block Success & Happiness - Bonus!

Training Exercise 7-1

Time to take stock of how much alignment you are already in. Sit comfortably and take a deep breath into your belly… and let it out. Let the next inhale come all of the way into your hips… and exhale. Relax your shoulders. Give yourself some quiet time to center in first.

Then when you are relaxed and centered, read the below questions and allow your deepest wisdom to answer frankly and honestly. DO NOT EDIT OR THINK – just let your inner voice be heard, take pen to paper, and circle your answer. You may be surprised at what happens.

Circle where you are at on this scale of 1-10.

1 = No not at all. 10 = 100% Yes.

1.   Do you give your body the proper food it needs to be fully nourished?

1   2   3   4   5   6   7   8   9   10

2.   Do you get enough rest?

1   2   3   4   5   6   7   8   9   10

3.   Do you get enough social time?

1   2   3   4   5   6   7   8   9   10

4.   Are your thoughts about yourself encouraging and kind?

1   2   3   4   5   6   7   8   9   10

5.   Do your words reflect the real appreciation you feel for your body?

1   2   3   4   5   6   7   8   9   10

6.   Do you get enough exercise to feel fit?

1   2   3   4   5   6   7   8   9   10

7.   Is there enough romance in your love-life?

1   2   3   4   5   6   7   8   9   10

8.   Do you feel valued and fairly compensated in your job?

1   2   3   4   5   6   7   8   9   10

9.   Are you willing to make amends with people you have wronged?

1   2   3   4   5   6   7   8   9   10

10.   Are you willing to forgive yourself?

1   2   3   4   5   6   7   8   9   10

11.   Are you willing to let yourself feel healthy, even if you are sick or injured?

1   2   3   4   5   6   7   8   9   10

12.   Is your home a safe, clean, calm haven?

1   2   3   4   5   6   7   8   9   10

13.   Does your work feel satisfying?

1   2   3   4   5   6   7   8   9   10

14.   Do you have enough fun with your kids – or if you don't have kids, do you have enough playtime?

1   2   3   4   5   6   7   8   9   10

15.   Do you have a habit of putting your physical needs first on your list?

1   2   3   4   5   6   7   8   9   10

16. Do you feel positive about your future?

1   2   3   4   5   6   7   8   9   10

17. Do you drink enough water every day? (1/2 of your body weight in pounds in ounces. For example: if you weigh 150 lbs divide by 2 = 75 ounces of water.)

1   2   3   4   5   6   7   8   9   10

18. Is feeling good a priority?

1   2   3   4   5   6   7   8   9   10

19. Is the way you live your life a reflection of your values?

1   2   3   4   5   6   7   8   9   10

(Ok, some of those questions aren't directly about your body, but each one of them effects your health in some way and I wanted to give you a chance to have a broader view of what health across the board looks like in your life.)

Tally your health vibe score to see where you are at:

180 – 190 - Health Vibe Superstar: You feel healthy all of the time, no matter what life throws at you. You radiate health and well being and others feel better just by being around you. Keep your daily health vibe practices going & remember to let others support you - or you know what happens, your health vibe drops!

155 – 179 - Health Vibe Rock star: You are able to feel healthy most of the time. There is stillroom to supercharge your health vibe, so keep practicing and be sure to get the extra support you need!

100 – 154 - Health Vibe Dancer: You are able to feel healthy sometimes, and the good news is that you are on your way to feeling much better! Keep up your health vibe training practices and be sure to get the extra support you need.

70 – 99 - Health Vibe Newbie: You are on your way to feeling healthier and more energized every day. Keep on practicing supercharging your health vibe and be sure to get the extra support you need.

19 – 69 - Health Vibe Red Alert: Ok, I'm officially worried about you. It's time to allow yourself to start feeling better. Go through this workbook again and participate fully in each training exercise. Be sure to get lots of outer world support from your healing team. Surround yourself with people that care about you. Do not go it alone, it is just too hard and you need an extra boost of energy to get you to supercharge your health vibe and feel better.

From your above answers you can clearly see what areas of your life you need to bring yourself into better centered alignment. This is a great indicator of where you need to supercharge your health vibe and take action to make changes - and always remember to get support from your healing team!

Training Exercise 7-2

Need to supercharge your Health Vibe Score or keep your score high? Time to write out an action plan. Refer back to the exercises in this book and schedule time in your calendar to do the ones that will help you supercharge your health vibe in your low score areas. Need to take some bold outer world actions? Bring yourself to centered alignment, hear your own wisdom, get support, and get out there in the world and take bold action to get it done!!

Keep it going – do this course over and over again to supercharge your health vibe and gain the inner strength to make the outer world changes you deserve!!

Training Exercise 7-3

You've made it to the final exercise of the Supercharge Your health Vibe Training - congratulations!

I'm having the best year of my life so far! Why? Because the first thing I do every morning is bring myself into centered alignment with my highest good. Remember how I used to align my energy with that of my imaginary romantic partner before getting out of bed and then one day he appeared? Well now I wake up every morning and the first thing I usually say to myself is, "I accept and love myself as I am." That is a great way to stop judgments and mean trash talk before it even starts!

Then I affirm: "My body is healthy and I feel great! I center and align myself with my highest good and get everything done today that needs to get done." And I mean everything: exercise, eating well, work, serving my clients, phone calls, socializing, which road to take... you name it. If it needs to get done it does. If it didn't get done, IT OBVIOUSLY DIDN'T NEED TO HAPPEN. I repeat that mantra throughout the day to make sure I stay on track and listen to my body and inner needs, so that my highest good is always guiding me. Because it knows better than I do - I'll skip meals and work myself into the ground unless I'm aligned first!

This trick allows me to be super productive, without burning myself out or being hard on myself. It allows me to respect my body and my relationships – because health and love come first for me! And yes, I still keep a successful career going, but not by sacrificing my health or my man. Now I trust that everything I do and everything I don't do is what needed to happen – and I let go of whatever I thought I "should" do. I stay strong and powerful throughout the whole workday and have more fun, nourishment, and rest when I need it.

Another great alignment statement is, "I'm in the perfect place at the perfect time." I love that one, especially when I'm sick or injured. It's really powerful.

Go ahead and plan what you are going to say and feel last thing before you go to sleep and first thing in the morning when you awake.

Before falling asleep I think and feel

_____

_____

Upon waking up I think and feel

_____

_____

Excellent! Now you are set to program yourself first thing in the morning and last thing at night. I do this every morning and night of my life. On the off chance I forget, I feel kind of lost in the morning and wander around until I get myself back into centered alignment with my highest good!

Want to know one of my little embarrassing secrets that really works to supercharge my health vibe? I'm a terrible singer and a goofy dancer, but if I sing a bouncy tune in my head or put on some music and shake my booty a bit – I FEEL SO MUCH BETTER IT IS AMAZING. As I am sitting here writing this workbook I am dancing in my seat. Yup, I'm all wiggly as I'm typing and I keep smiling because I don't really know the words and I'm kind of butchering the tune and repeating the same part over again, but it is working to supercharge my health vibe, so I'm doing it! And that is a key to healing. You've got to be WILLING to heal. You've got to be willing to look silly, feel happy for no reason, and let go of the baggage that has held you back for years. Just BE WILLING, COMMIT to doing your training exercises, get SUPPORT, and you will supercharge your health vibe.

Here is a very personal, very extreme example of getting into centered alignment.

I'm sharing it with you only because I intuit that some of you need to hear this level of my message to really get the importance of why centered alignment matters so much. Spring of 2014 my neighbor had a violent outburst and my man and I suddenly decided to move out of our home. We didn't feel safe staying there, and even though we lived in an affordable apartment in the middle of our favorite neighborhood of Los Feliz, our safety came first and we decided to move out.

We knew it was going to be stressful and we didn't want it to negatively impact our relationship, so we made a vow that we would not take out our fear or frustration on each other.

Even though we were utterly unprepared, we immediately rallied all of our friends and allies to pack our entire home and move out in just one day. We didn't know where we would end up and it was a very scary venture. But, we knew in our hearts that we were doing the right thing and that we would get through this together.

After we suddenly moved out, a generous kind friend gave us a place to stay while we were looking for a new home. 6 weeks later we were living in a new, luxury, huge, home at a price we could afford. We each had our own home office and felt incredibly grateful. AND, as fantastic as that apartment was and as in alignment as it was for us when we got it, we knew we would not be there long. We moved out after a year, but didn't find a new apartment in time and had to put everything in storage and spend the summer staying with awesome friends and subletting.

Sure, it was not convenient, but we knew we were in alignment with our next home and we just kept scouring the city and attracting it by vibrating at the frequency of us feeling happy in a home we love.

Now we live in the BEST home we've ever had together! It is exactly where we wanted up in the hills, has a great view, spacious, high ceilings, 2 fire places, a Jacuzzi tub, and we can walk to restaurants right down the street. We love it here! And, due to changing circumstances, we may have to move again next year, but we are staying in centered alignment and grateful for each wonderful home that comes our way.

Here is the secret truth I'm going to reveal to you, we hadn't been in alignment with that first Los Feliz apartment for a long time. We LOVED the location and the price and we were full of gratitude to be able to live there, that is why we stayed so long, but the quality of the building and management was very low and there wasn't enough space for us to comfortably live and work. It didn't match our love, money, or health vibe to stay living there nor did it match our centered alignment.

When you are not in centered alignment with your highest good, something always comes along and happens to try to FORCE YOU into alignment with your highest good. That most often happens in a disruptive way.

Over the last 23 years of helping people heal I have seen something happen over and over again; when people do not take good enough care of their health and well being, they often get sick or injured to a point that forces them to stay in bed and receive care. If they are stuck in a rut with finances, a traumatic unexpected expense happens. Or if they are out of alignment with their love life, a sudden upset or break up occurs. Can you think of a time when any of those ever happened to you? Is it happening to you now? Maybe you didn't recognize it as such until you got through this course, but I bet now you can see the link between what is going on in your life, the vibrations you are giving off, and whether or not you are in centered alignment!

Centered Alignment first allows Health
to infuse every area of your life.

CHAPTER 8 - ROUND UP

Let's take stock of how you have already begun to supercharge your health vibe:

1.   You've shifted health beliefs that were holding you back and your thoughts towards your body are now kind and loving.

2.   You understand that needs are natural.

3.   You value your own self worth.

4.   You've made amends and are willing to forgive yourself.

5.   You've opened the flow of giving and receiving.

6.   You've gained appreciation for your body.

7.   You've activated your inner health magnet and can attract more vitality to you.

8.   You speak words of love & healing to yourself and others.

9.   You've shifted to an attitude of gratitude.

10.   You allow yourself to feel healthy now.

11.   You've gotten into centered alignment!

12.   You've scheduled a Health Vibe action plan in your calendar!

If you want to feel healthier and more energized, then regularly practice everything you learned throughout this Supercharge Your Health Vibe training.

Don't stop. Do an exercise every day – I do! That is how I keep supercharging my health vibe!

The issues I discuss in this book are what I had to deal with to open up my health channels - and I continue to improve. I've learned that the more abundance, love, and health I notice all around me and let myself feel, the stronger my healing capabilities have become, and the more I can help others to heal.

My health vibe keeps improving steadily over time and shows itself in all kinds of ways.

- I feel healthy and energized all day long.

- I rarely ever get sick.

- All organic delicious food!

- I delight my body with all natural products with no sulfites or perfumes.

- My home is clean and calm, so I feel relaxed and healthy here.

- I have a great healing team and I get massages, acupuncture, therapy, healings and chiropractic care.

- I take the right supplements for my body.

- I keep up on new healing modalities and neuroscience breakthroughs.

- Pedicures 2x a month to show appreciation to my feet that have endured 2 surgeries each.

- People tell me they feel good just hanging out with me.

- 49 years old 5'6" 125#.

- Strong enough to hike or dance for hours and feel great!

- I've let go of people, food, and things that weren't healing for me.

- I'm so overflowing with vitality that I attract wonderful clients and feel excited to go to work each day.

Look back to exercise #1. How have those things on your list improved? Don't be hard on yourself if they haven't improved as much as you want them to YET. That just shows that you need to keep practicing supercharging your health vibe.

Sometimes it takes hours and sometimes years to be able to sustain certain energy frequencies. Remember, it took me 2 years to get my love vibe strong enough for this awesome relationship I'm now in!

And remember, you don't have to go it alone. I see so many women struggle by either trying to do everything all by themselves, or by thinking they can't stand on their own two feet. Both ends of that spectrum are painful! If you were meant to go it alone, there would only be one person walking the planet. So, never feel ashamed if you need help. You deserve to get the support that you truly need to transform your life in every way you want.

The Happy Woman Academy is full of generous caring women who have so much love to give, always feel free to reach out and ask for help. We love being here for each other, including YOU! We'll give you a system, support, motivation, and accountability in supercharging your money, love, and health vibe.

Just connect with www.TheHappyWomanAcademy.com to see when our next virtual course and live event or party is.

Let's all keep practicing supercharging our health vibe together so we can keep supercharging the health vibe on our planet and help everybody to feel the energy, health, and vitality they deserve.

I'm so pleased that you made it through this training and I sincerely hope that you keep practicing because I know how well it worked for me, my clients, and it will work for you. I look forward to hearing the great stories of how you have supercharged your health vibe!

With love, health, and gratitude,
Elizabeth

CHAPTER 9 - RESOURCES

If you are in Los Angeles, come on our Happy Woman Hike on the first Saturday of every month! Just enter www.TheHappyWomanAcademy.com

If you'd like to receive 1-1 mentorship with me, you can apply for a Best Next Step Call at bit.ly/bestnextstep. If you qualify, we'll have a dedicated in depth conversation to discover the best next step on your healing path.

If you are a man, get the community you need here: DaleThomasVaughn.com.

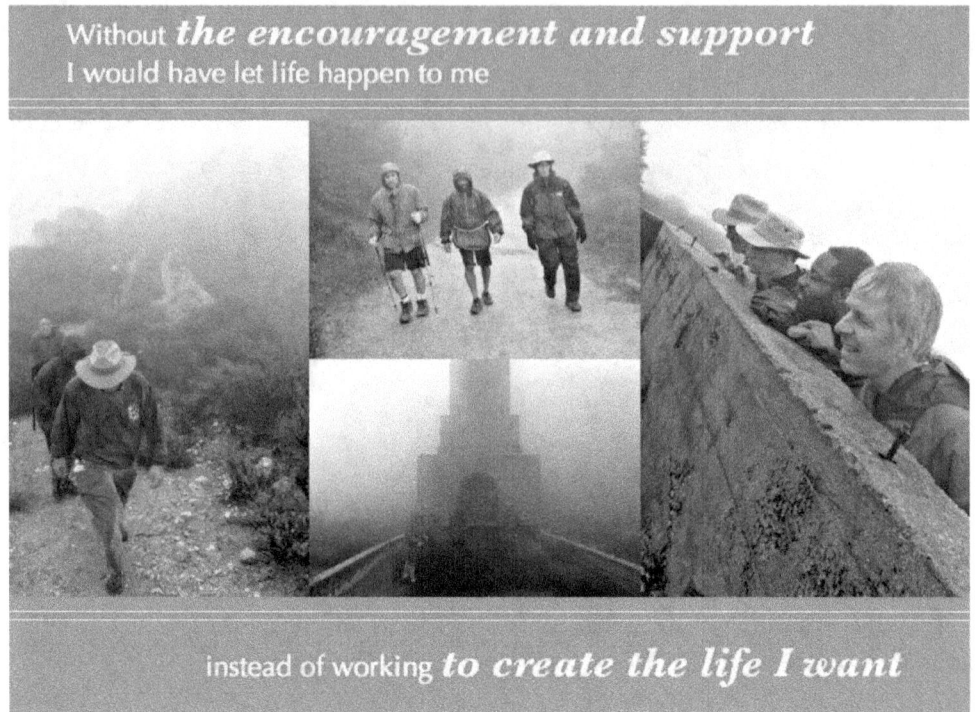

Photos by Ken Morris (Glitch.photography) and Eric Beteille (PedestrianPhotographer.com).

ALSO BY ELIZABETH MENZEL

Supercharge Your Money Vibe!

WOMEN'S HEALTH BEST-SELLER

Get ready to learn the exact ways I quadrupled my financial income by changing my poverty consciousness to prosperity consciousness as well as how I improved my relationship with money – all while keeping my integrity and working less hours - so that you can do the same for yourself.

Supercharge Your Love Vibe!

WOMEN'S HEALTH BEST-SELLER

Get ready to learn the exact ways I attracted the man of my dreams by changing my broken heart into the well spring of love it's meant to be. As well as how I improved my relationship with my family, my emotions, my body, humanity, and romance, so that you can do the same for yourself.

The 10-Minute Memoir

BEST-SELLER

This book came from a deep heartfelt desire to know the stories of my family. Write Your Memoir In Just 10 Minutes A Day With This Easy Q&A Journal

ABOUT ELIZABETH

Elizabeth Menzel is a certified Brennan Healing Science practitioner and serves as a speaker, best selling author, Happy Woman Mentor, and she's the founder of the award winning Happy Woman Academy. Her books and programs focus on ending the cycle of sacrifice, sabotage, and neglect so that women can enjoy massive success in their career, health, and love life.

She uses proven neuroscience and physics based healing systems and has facilitated thousands of transformations over the last 23 years. Her live events & Happiness Training Programs teach busy women of all ages powerful "on the go" ways to heal their body, invigorate their romance, and boost their career – so they can receive more money while enjoying life more fully! She's on a mission to teach 1,000,000 women "The Happy Woman Formula" by 2020.

The mission of the Happy Woman Academy is to provide women with a safe and sacred space to learn how to easily receive more love, health, and money by using proven science based healing systems and the power of communion and laughter.

The vision of the Happy Woman Academy is to restore the Feminine to her rightful place of honor & value next to the Masculine in society, thereby restoring harmonic balance to humanity, the earth, & nature. Big vision I know, but it's the one I've got.

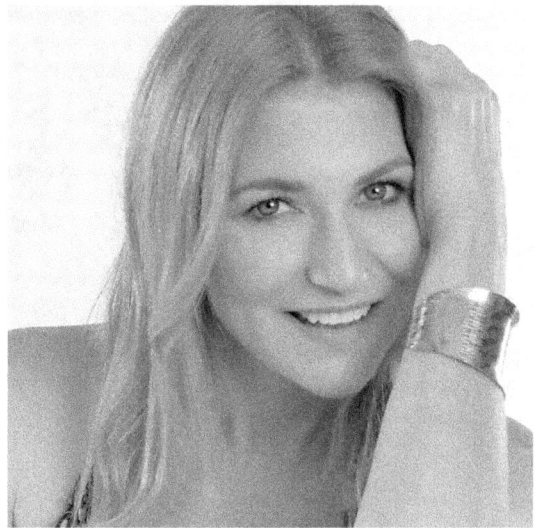

CONNECT WITH ME

Visit www.TheHappyWomanAcademy.com/quiz
And take the 30 second quiz to find out the
#1 way you Sabotage Your Success & Happiness

AND

Visit the Happy Woman Academy on Facebook at
https://www.facebook.com/TheHappyWomanAcademy/

AND

I love hearing from my readers, so please feel free to
leave a positive review on my Amazon Author page
at bit.ly/AmazonAuthorElizabethMenzel

BIBLIOGRAPHY

[1] Wijk, Roeland Van. "An Introduction to Human Biophoton Emission." *National Center for Biotechnology Information*. U.S. National Library of Medicine, 12 Apr. 2005. Web. 21 Mar. 2015.

[2] William Walker Atkinson. Thought Vibration or the Law of Attraction. Advanced Thought Publishing. 1906

[3] Tan, Enoch. "Secrets of Mind and Reality." Nature of Vibration in the Spiritual Dimension. MindReality.com. Web. 21 Mar. 2015.

[4] Bergeisen, Michael. "The Neuroscience of Happiness." *The Neuroscience of Happiness*. Berkeley College, 23 Sept. 2010. Web. 21 Mar. 2015.
Journal of Homosexuality, Vol. 45(1) 2003

[5] Turner, Ashley. "How Meditation Changes Your Brain Frequency." *MindBodyGreen*. MindBodyGreen.com, 5 Feb. 2014. Web. 21 Mar. 2015.

[6] Lagopoulos et al. Increased Theta and Alpha EEG Activity During Nondirective Meditation. The Journal of Alternative and Complementary Medicine, 2009; 15 (11): 1187 DOI: 10.1089/acm.2009.0113

[7] Hurley, Dan. "Grandma's Experiences Leave a Mark on Your Genes." *Discover Magazine*. DiscoverMagazine.com, 11 June 2013. Web. 21 Mar. 2015.
Nature Neuroscience 7, 847 - 854 (2004)

[8] Jornal de Pediatria - Vol. 80, No.2(Suppl), 2004

[9] The Journal of Neuroscience7 *June 2006, 26(23): 6314-6317*

[10] Szalavitz, Maia. "Reality Check: Why Some Brains Can't Tell Real From Imagined | TIME.com." *Time.com*. Time, 5 Oct. 2011. Web. 21 Mar. 2015.

[11] The Journal of Neuroscience, October 5, 2011 31(40):14308–14313

[12] NeuroReport 11:1581±1585 & 2000 Lippincott Williams & Wilkins

[13] I include motherhood as a full time job and admirable career choice.

[14] Human Diseases and Conditions, http://www.KidsHealth.org
Neil Izenberg, M.D.

[15] Psychoneuroendocrinology. 2013 Mar;38(3):348-55. doi: 10.1016/j.psyneuen. 2012.06.011. Epub 2012 Jul 15. Indian J Exp Biol. 2008 May;46(5):345-52. Author: I. S. Rattan, Suresh